COMPLETE GUIDE TO JOINT REPLACEMENT SURGERY

Comprehensive Handbook To Recovery, Benefits, Risks, And Rehabilitation For Hip, Knee, And Shoulder Procedures

DR. BRUNO HORAN

Copyright © 2023 by Dr. Bruno Horan

All rights reserved. Except for brief quotations embodied in critical reviews and certain other noncommercial uses permitted by copyright law, no part of this publication may be reproduced, distributed, or transmitted in any form or by any means, Including photocopying, recording, or other electronic or mechanical methods, without the prior written permission of the publisher.

Disclaimer:

The information provided in this book, is intended for general informational purposes only and should not be considered as professional advice.

The author has made every effort to ensure the accuracy of the information presented. However, readers are advised to consult with a qualified healthcare professional before attempting any herbal remedies or making significant changes to their wellness routine. Individual health conditions vary, and what may be suitable for one person may not be appropriate for another.

It is important to note that the author is not in any endorsement deal, partnership, or affiliation with any organization, brand, or company mentioned in this book. Any references to specific products or services are based on the author's personal experience or general knowledge and do not imply an endorsement or promotion of those products or services

Contents

CHAPTER ONE 13
JOINT REPLACEMENT SURGERY TYPES 13
An Overview Of Replacements For The Knee, Hip, Shoulders, And Elbow 13

A Comparative Analysis Of Surgical Methods 15

Pros And Cons Of Every Category 17

Selection Criteria For The Appropriate Surgery ... 18

Getting Mentally And Physically Ready For Surgery 19

CHAPTER TWO 21
SETTING UP FOR SURGERY TO REPLACE A JOINT 21
Assessment And Examination Of Medicines 21

Exercises And Rehabilitation Prior To Surgery 22

Mental Readiness And Guidance 22

Nutritional Advice Prior To Surgery 23

Setting Up Support And Home Care 23

CHAPTER THREE 25
THE HOSPITAL STAY AND THE DAY OF SURGERY 25
A Comprehensive Guide For Surgery Day 25

Options And Dangers Of Anesthesia 26

What Takes Place During Surgery......................27
Procedures In The Recovery Room After Surgery 28
First Hospitalization And Surveillance 28

CHAPTER FOUR 31
REPAY AND RESUMMATION 31
Quick Post-Operative Care 31
Physical Rehabilitation Exercises And Plans 32
Techniques For Pain Management 33
Controlling Inflammation And Swelling...............34
Tracking Development And Modifying Operations
....34

CHAPTER FIVE 37
POSSIBLE RISKS AND COMPLICATIONS 37
Typical Post-Surgical Complications 37
Management And Prevention Of Infections.........39
Prevention And Risks Of Blood Clots 41
Problems With Implants And Long-Term Issues..43
Indications Of Difficulties: When To Contact Your
Physician 44

CHAPTER SIX...47
AFTER A JOINT REPLACEMENT: LIFE 47

Getting Used To The New Joint Motion And
   Function 47
   Going Back To Work And Daily Activities 48
   Tips For Long-Term Maintenance And Care 50
   Modifications To Lifestyle For Joint Health..........51
   Athletics And Exercise Following Rehabilitation ...52
CHAPTER SEVEN 55
   OTHER MEDICAL SUGGESTIONS AND THERAPIES 55
   Alternatives To Surgery For Joint Pain 55
   Alternatives To Physical Therapy 55
   Methods In Regenerative Medicine 56
   Complementary Medicine For Bone Health 57
CHAPTER EIGHT 59
   IMPACT ON EMOTIONS AND PSYCHOLOGY 59
   Handling Emotional Difficulties 59
   Options For Counseling And Support Systems 60
   Post-Surgery Mental Health Considerations 60
   Community Resources And Peer Assistance........61
   Keeping An Optimistic Attitude 62
CHAPTER NINE 63
   COMMON QUESTIONS AND ANSWERS 63

Timetable For Recuperation And Expectations 65

Going Back To Work And Daily Schedule............66

Mobility And Travel Considerations 67

Observational Care And Medical Visits................68

Meeting The Needs For Social And Family Support 69

CONCERNING THIS BOOK

For anyone planning or currently undergoing joint replacement surgery, this extensive guide titled "Joint Replacement Surgery" is an invaluable resource. Given the importance of joints for movement and day-to-day functioning, it is imperative to comprehend the nuances of joint health. The book opens with a thorough examination of joint replacement surgery, highlighting the procedure's significance in improving the quality of life for those with incapacitating joint problems.

It begins by exploring the foundations of joint health and identifying common disorders that frequently require surgery. The book provides readers with the necessary information to make well-informed judgments about their treatment options by highlighting the advantages and hazards of joint replacement surgery. By providing a comparative examination of several surgical procedures for elbow, shoulder, hip, and knee replacements, the book gives readers the information they need to make the best decision for their particular situation.

Thorough planning is necessary for joint replacement surgery, both emotionally and physically. All aspects are addressed to guarantee a seamless transition into the surgical process, ranging from pre-surgery rehabilitation exercises to dietary advice and psychological preparation.

An extensive road map for what to anticipate both during and after surgery is provided with thorough insights into anesthesia alternatives, surgical techniques, and immediate post-surgery care.

Comprehensive coverage is provided for the crucial stages of recovery and rehabilitation, which center on controlling pain, lowering inflammation, and avoiding complications with professional assistance.

The book also focuses on life following joint replacement, providing helpful advice on how to resume everyday activities, adapt to new joint functions, and preserve long-term joint health.

The handbook addresses psychological and emotional issues and offers coping mechanisms for dealing with difficulties that arise after surgery, stressing the value of support networks and mental health services.

In order to provide clarity on recovery periods, follow-up care, and lifestyle adaptations required for sustained joint health and mobility, it finishes with a full analysis of common issues and FAQs.

"Joint Replacement Surgery" is a lifeline for people starting along the path to better mobility, freedom, and general well-being, not just a guidebook.

CHAPTER ONE

JOINT REPLACEMENT SURGERY TYPES

An Overview Of Replacements For The Knee, Hip, Shoulders, And Elbow

The treatment of severe joint problems like arthritis has been revolutionized by joint replacement procedures, which have helped many people restore mobility and reduce discomfort. The most popular kinds are replacements for the knee, hip, shoulder, and elbow.

Each focuses on particular joints where damage or degeneration has significantly affected day-to-day functioning.

Knee Replacement: Artificial materials are used to replace damaged knee joint surfaces in this treatment. For people with severe arthritis or joint injuries that impair stability and mobility, it's frequently advised.

Patients can benefit from increased range of motion and less discomfort by having the damaged portions of their knee resurfaced, which will greatly enhance their quality of life.

Hip Replacement: To treat diseases like osteoarthritis or fractures that seriously limit hip joint function, hip replacements are frequently carried out.

In order to replace the damaged bone and cartilage, prosthetic parts that mimic the motion and stability of the native hip joint are surgically inserted. This technique has a reputation for successfully reducing pain and improving movement.

Shoulder Replacement: For people with severe arthritis or irreversible rotator cuff damage, shoulder joint replacement is a less common but very successful treatment option.

It entails using prosthetic components to replace the injured shoulder joint elements, resulting in less pain and smoother mobility. Range of motion can be greatly increased and shoulder function can be restored with shoulder replacements.

Elbow Replacement: Disorders like severe arthritis or fractures that affect the function of the elbow joint are treated with elbow joint replacement surgery.

During the treatment, artificial components that replicate the mechanics of the elbow joint found in nature are used to replace broken bone and cartilage. The purpose of this procedure is to improve overall arm function by reducing discomfort and regaining elbow movement.

A Comparative Analysis Of Surgical Methods

Depending on the patient's condition and the structure of the joint, different surgical techniques are used for different types of joint replacement surgery.

Different strategies, such as minimally invasive procedures and open surgery, may be employed by surgeons.

Conventional Open Surgery: To reach the joint during a traditional joint replacement procedure, a bigger incision is created.

This gives the surgeon clear access and view to remove diseased tissue and precisely place the prosthetic components. Even if it works, the healing period and rehabilitation process are usually longer.

Minimally Invasive Surgery: To perform surgery with less damage to surrounding tissues, minimally invasive procedures make smaller incisions and use specialized instruments.

This method frequently results in quicker rehabilitation, less discomfort following surgery, and shorter recovery periods. However, depending on how complicated their illness is, not every patient may be a good fit.

Pros And Cons Of Every Category

Replacement of the Knee:

Advantages: Prolonged pain alleviation, increased mobility, and durable effects.

Cons: Higher risk of infection, longer time to heal, limited activity at first.

Replacement of the Hip:

Advantages: Significantly less discomfort, better hip function, and more range of motion.

Cons: Long healing time, possibility for leg length inequality, and dislocation risk.

Replacement of the Shoulders:

Advantages: Pain relief, increased range of motion, and better shoulder function.

Cons: Extended recovery, chance of nerve damage, and infection risk.

Replacement Elbow:

Advantages: Relieved pain, improved arm function, and restored elbow movement.

Cons: Possible component wear, infection risk, and occasionally restricted range of motion.

Selection Criteria For The Appropriate Surgery

Several considerations should be carefully evaluated before deciding to have joint replacement surgery:

Condition Severity: How severe is the arthritis or joint damage?

Health and Lifestyle: Recuperation and success are influenced by general health and degree of activity.

Patient Objectives: What is the anticipated level of pain alleviation and enhanced functionality?

Medical History: Current ailments and dangers associated with surgery.

Getting Mentally And Physically Ready For Surgery

Joint replacement surgery requires both mental and physical preparation:

Physical Preparation: performing activities to build muscle, keeping a healthy weight, and adhering to pre-operative instructions.

Mental Preparation: Comprehending the process, talking with medical professionals about any worries, and setting up the house for healing.

Every stage of the process, from knowing what kinds of operations are available to get ready for the operation, is essential to guaranteeing good results and a higher standard of living for patients having joint replacement surgery.

CHAPTER TWO

SETTING UP FOR SURGERY TO REPLACE A JOINT

Assessment And Examination Of Medicines

In order to evaluate your general health and establish if you are a good candidate for joint replacement surgery, a comprehensive medical evaluation and testing are necessary prior to the procedure.

A battery of tests, such as blood tests, imaging scans (MRIs or X-rays), and maybe an electrocardiogram (ECG) to assess heart function, will usually be performed by your doctor.

These examinations aid in the detection of any underlying illnesses that may have an impact on your recuperation or the procedure itself.

Exercises And Rehabilitation Prior To Surgery

It is essential to participate in pre-operative rehabilitation and exercises in order to maximize your physical state and improve the results of total joint replacement surgery.

Your medical staff might suggest particular activities designed to increase flexibility, strengthen the muscles surrounding the joint, and improve mobility in general. These workouts are crucial to your body's rehabilitation after surgery since they not only help your body get ready for the procedure.

Mental Readiness And Guidance

Just as crucial as the physical preparation for joint replacement surgery is the mental preparation. You can address any worries or anxieties you may have about the surgery and reduce anxiety by attending counseling sessions with a healthcare expert. An optimistic outlook and significant reduction in stress can be fostered by being aware of what to expect both during and after surgery, both of which are advantageous for healing.

Nutritional Advice Prior To Surgery

Before having joint replacement surgery, you can promote your general health and speed up the healing process by adhering to the recommended dietary instructions.

To maximize your nutritional status, your healthcare professional might suggest a well-balanced diet high in vitamins and minerals. Dietary changes, such as consuming more protein or less sodium, may be suggested in some circumstances in order to facilitate a quicker recovery after surgery.

Setting Up Support And Home Care

For a seamless recovery after joint replacement surgery, home and support care arrangements must be made in advance. This could entail making arrangements for help with everyday tasks like cleaning, meal preparation, and getting to and from doctor's appointments.

Making sure your house has the proper accommodations, like as raised toilet seats or railings, can help improve comfort and safety while you heal.

CHAPTER THREE

THE HOSPITAL STAY AND THE DAY OF SURGERY

A Comprehensive Guide For Surgery Day

You will first need to be at the hospital or surgical facility on the day of your joint replacement procedure, usually early in the morning.

You'll be led to a preoperative area where you'll change into a hospital gown after completing the required admittance paperwork.

Your medical history will be reviewed by nurses and other medical experts, who will also confirm the specifics of the treatment and make sure all essential arrangements have been made.

You will meet with the anesthesiologist to go over your alternatives for anesthesia after everything has been confirmed. There are two primary forms of anesthetic used in joint replacement surgery: regional and general.

While regional anesthesia, such as spinal or epidural anesthesia, numbs the lower half of your body while allowing you to remain aware, a general anesthetic will render you unconscious for the length of the surgery.

Options And Dangers Of Anesthesia

Selecting the appropriate anesthetic is essential for joint replacement surgery. Despite being used more frequently, general anesthetic has a marginally increased risk of side effects including nausea, vomiting, and allergic responses.

Throughout the process, your vital signs must be closely monitored as well. Conversely, regional anesthetic lowers the dangers and effectively relieves pain, although it may not be appropriate for everyone, particularly for people with specific medical conditions.

What Takes Place During Surgery

The orthopedic surgeon will start the surgery after the surgical team has prepped the operating room and you are under anesthesia.

Usually, an incision is made across the joint, diseased bone and cartilage are removed, and prosthetic parts composed of ceramic, metal, or plastic are placed in their place.

To maximize the joint replacement's lifetime and functionality, extra attention is taken to guarantee correct alignment and stability.

Advanced medical equipment and imaging technologies may be used throughout the procedure to help the surgeon precisely place the implants.

The entire procedure is carefully designed and carried out to efficiently relieve pain and restore joint function.

Procedures In The Recovery Room After Surgery

You will be brought to the recovery area, sometimes referred to as the post-anesthesia care unit (PACU), once the procedure is finished. Here, when you start to come out of anesthesia, medical professionals will keep a careful eye on your vital signs and general health. We'll start pain management techniques, such as IV drugs or nerve blocks, to make sure you're comfortable throughout this early stage of rehabilitation.

First Hospitalization And Surveillance

You will be moved to a hospital room to start your postoperative treatment and rehabilitation after spending time in the recovery room.

Your overall health, the particular joint that has been replaced, and how well you respond to treatment are some of the variables that may affect how long you stay in the hospital. Physical therapists and nurses will work closely with you during this period to help you restore mobility, manage pain, and avoid problems like infections or blood clots.

Regular monitoring of your surgery site, vital signs, and overall recovery progress will be carried out throughout your hospital stay to make sure you are healing appropriately and reaching discharge goals. The following stage of therapy, which frequently takes place at home or in a specialist rehabilitation facility, depends on careful care to help you recover successfully.

CHAPTER FOUR

REPAY AND RESUMMATION

Quick Post-Operative Care

The priority after joint replacement surgery changes to make sure the patient recovers well and avoids problems.

It's likely that you'll spend some time in the recovery area, where medical professionals will keep an eye on your vital signs and make sure you're at ease.

Depending on your individual needs, you will be transferred to either a standard hospital room or a rehabilitation center after being cleared by your medical team.

It's critical that you carefully follow the advice of your healthcare team at this initial stage. This includes controlling discomfort, using prescription drugs, and keeping an eye on any drainage or wound care requirements.

To minimize stiffness and improve circulation, you can be urged to begin with mild motions; nevertheless, you should avoid putting too much weight or force on the recently replaced joint.

Physical Rehabilitation Exercises And Plans

During the healing process following joint replacement surgery, physical therapy is essential. A physical therapist will carefully collaborate with you to create a customized workout program soon after surgery. These exercises are intended to promote appropriate healing while helping the joint regain its strength, flexibility, and range of motion.

In order to prevent stiffness and minimize swelling, the first part of therapy may concentrate on passive exercises and moderate movements.

The level of intensity and complexity of exercises will rise progressively as your recuperation advances. Activities to enhance balance, coordination, and functional motions relevant to your everyday life may fall under this category.

Techniques For Pain Management

After joint replacement surgery, pain control is crucial to a comfortable recovery. Your healthcare team will use a mix of drugs and methods to minimize side effects and manage pain levels. To treat acute pain, painkillers might first be used orally or intravenously.

Your healthcare practitioner may give oral pain medicines and suggest non-drug therapies like heat therapy or ice packs when you go from the hospital to home care.

It's critical to be transparent with your healthcare team about your pain thresholds so that any necessary modifications to your pain management strategy can be implemented.

Controlling Inflammation And Swelling

Following joint replacement surgery, swelling and inflammation are typical and are treated using a variety of strategies to aid in healing and comfort. Early on, edema can be lessened by elevating the injured leg, using compression clothing, and using cold packs. Your healthcare staff can also suggest particular workouts and motions to enhance blood flow and lessen fluid accumulation near the joint.

Tracking Development And Modifying Operations

Following joint replacement surgery, you will need to schedule follow-up consultations with your healthcare team to monitor your progress. They will evaluate your strength, range of motion, and general healing process during these sessions. To assess the location and functionality of the replacement joint, X-rays or other imaging studies might be carried out.

Your healthcare practitioner will modify your physical therapy regimen and activity level based on your progress.

They might offer instructions on how to resume daily activities including driving, walking, and climbing stairs as well as how to gradually increase weight-bearing activities. Adhering to these guidelines contributes to the triumphant recuperation and enduring performance of your recently acquired joint.

CHAPTER FIVE

POSSIBLE RISKS AND COMPLICATIONS

Typical Post-Surgical Complications

It's important to be aware of any issues that may emerge during the healing period after joint replacement surgery. Infections, blood clots, implant malfunctions, and indications of more serious consequences that would necessitate emergency care are common difficulties.

Infection: Following surgery, one of the biggest worries is infection. Fever or chills, together with symptoms like increased redness, swelling, or warmth near the surgery site, could be signs of an infection. To avoid problems, prompt medical examination and antibiotic therapy are essential.

Blood Clots: The development of blood clots is an additional danger following joint replacement surgery.

These may begin as deep vein thrombosis in the legs and possibly spread to the lungs (pulmonary embolism). Early mobilization, compression stockings, and occasionally blood-thinning drugs are methods used to avoid blood clots.

Implant Issues: From time to time, issues may arise with the joint implant. This may involve gradual wear, dislocation, or loosening.

Early detection and management of these disorders can be facilitated by regular follow-up meetings with your surgeon and monitoring the joint's function.

Long-Term Considerations: Although joint replacement surgery has a high success rate, there are some long-term things to think about. The prosthetic joint may deteriorate over time and need revision surgery. Maintaining an active lifestyle, controlling weight, and according to your surgeon's instructions can all help the implant last longer.

Management And Prevention Of Infections

Keeping Infections At Bay Following Surgery

One of the most important aspects of joint replacement post-surgery care is infection prevention. Surgical teams employ stringent measures to reduce the risk of infection during the procedure, including the use of sterile methods and the administration of antibiotics. Furthermore, patients are recommended to:

Taking Care of the Incision: It's crucial to maintain a dry and clean surgical site. Observe the wound care recommendations provided by your surgeon, including when to take a shower and change dressings.

Keep an Eye Out for Infection-Related Symptoms: Pay close attention to any signs of growing discomfort, redness, swelling, or drainage from the incision. Chills or fever can also be signs of an infection and should be treated right away.

Complete Antibiotics: If you are prescribed antibiotics, make sure to take them exactly as prescribed by your physician.

It helps stop the growth of resistant germs and guarantees effective treatment when antibiotics are taken to the end of their recommended course.

Handling Infections Should They Emerge

Even with precautions taken, infections can still happen following joint replacement surgery. Typically, treatment entails:

Antibiotics: It's critical to give antibiotics according to the infection kind. In the event of a more serious infection, intravenous antibiotics may be used instead of oral antibiotics.

Surgical Intervention: To completely clear an infection, it may be required to surgically drain the infection or even remove the implant. Based on your unique circumstances, your healthcare team will decide on the best course of action.

Recovery and Rehabilitation: Healing from an infection could make recovery from it take longer. To get the best recovery results, physical treatment and careful monitoring of the joint function are necessary.

Prevention And Risks Of Blood Clots

Knowing the Risks of Blood Clots

There's a chance of blood clots after joint replacement surgery, especially in the leg veins. If these clots come loose and go to the lungs, they could be harmful. The following variables raise the chance of clotting:

Surgical Procedure: The act of doing surgery itself may momentarily alter blood flow, which raises the risk of clotting.

Immobilization: Following surgery, a limited range of motion might impede blood circulation and increase the risk of clot formation.

Medical History: Smoking, obesity, blood clots in the past, and certain drugs can further raise the risk of clotting.

How to Avoid Blood Clots

Your medical team might suggest the following to lower the risk of blood clots:

Early Mobilization: Following surgery, getting up and moving as soon as possible enhances blood flow and lowers the chance of clotting.

Compression Stockings: By keeping blood from collecting in the legs, compression stockings can help lower the risk of blood clot formation.

Medication: To lower the risk of clotting, blood-thinning drugs like aspirin or heparin may be administered for a while following surgery.

Problems With Implants And Long-Term Issues

Prospects for Joint Implants in the Long Run

Even though joint replacement surgery greatly reduces pain and increases mobility, there are a number of factors that affect how long an implant lasts:

Wear and Tear: With repeated use, the artificial joint may eventually deteriorate. The joint may become unstable or loose as a result of this wear.

Activity Level: Excessive weight-bearing or high-impact activities might limit the implant's lifespan by accelerating deterioration.

Frequent Monitoring: To keep an eye on the implant's performance and identify any early indicators of wear or possible problems, schedule routine follow-up visits with your surgeon.

Handling Problems with Implants

It's critical to speak with your healthcare physician as soon as possible if you experience any issues with the joint implant, such as pain, decreased range of motion, or instability. Possible course of treatment options include:

Revision Surgery: To replace the worn-out implant or treat issues like loosening or infection, revision surgery might be required in some circumstances.

Physical treatment: Physical treatment can improve the longevity of the implant by strengthening the surrounding muscles and maintaining joint function.

Indications Of Difficulties: When To Contact Your Physician

Identifying Symptoms That Need Medical Attention

Certain post-joint replacement symptoms need to be seen by a doctor right once in order to stop issues from getting worse. Among them are:

Severe Pain: Pain that comes on suddenly or gets worse and is not better with medicine could be a sign of an infection, blood clot, or implant complications.

Swelling or Redness: Profound swelling, redness, or warmth in the vicinity of the surgical site may indicate an infection or inflammation that has to be investigated.

Fever or chills: Fever more than 100.4°F (38°C) or chills may be signs of an infection and should be evaluated by a doctor every once.

Breathing Problems: Chest pain, shortness of breath, or blood in the cough may indicate a pulmonary embolism, which is a blood clot in the lungs that needs to be treated very once.

Changes in Mobility: You should notify your healthcare physician right away if you experience any unexpected changes in joint function, such as instability or difficulties moving the joint.

Persistent Drainage: If you observe a persistent discharge or drainage from the surgery site, you should get checked out by a doctor since it might be an infection.

General Concerns: Believe your gut. Please don't hesitate to ask your healthcare staff for advice if you have any questions about your recuperation or if you observe any strange symptoms.

CHAPTER SIX

AFTER A JOINT REPLACEMENT: LIFE

Getting Used To The New Joint Motion And Function

One of the most important stages of recovery following joint replacement surgery is getting used to the new movement and functionality of your joint.

It's typical to feel stiff and uncomfortable around the surgery site for a while as your body adjusts to the prosthetic joint.

During this time, physical therapy is crucial because it progressively helps you rebuild your strength, flexibility, and range of motion.

Your therapist will lead you through exercises intended to increase muscular strength and joint mobility during physical therapy sessions. These workouts are designed just for you and will assist you in regaining the capacity to carry out daily tasks more easily. Your joint's range of motion will get better as you go along, enabling more fluid and natural movements.

To ensure the best possible recovery, it's critical that you do as your therapist instructs and stick to the suggested workout schedule.

As you progressively regain confidence in using your new joint, consistency, and patience are essential. You'll discover that tasks like walking, climbing stairs, and bending get simpler and less painful with time.

Going Back To Work And Daily Activities

After joint replacement surgery, resuming everyday activities and employment necessitates careful planning and a gradual return to tasks.

At first, you might require help with specific tasks, like driving or doing housework. During this changeover phase, it's critical to pay attention to your body and refrain from overexerting yourself.

Consult your healthcare team to make sure you're physically prepared for the demands of your job before going back to work.

Depending on your line of work, you might need to alter to facilitate your recovery by changing your workspace or timetable.

Additionally, your employer might offer assistance through flexible work schedules or ergonomic evaluations.

As you get back into your normal routine, give priority to the things that will help your new joint recover and avoid tension.

If your doctor advises you to use assistive technology, do so to lessen the strain on your joints when walking or lifting things.

You'll feel more confident and at ease returning to your regular obligations if you gradually increase your activity level and pay attention to your body's cues.

Tips For Long-Term Maintenance And Care

Taking a proactive stance when it comes to long-term care is necessary to preserve the longevity and well-being of your new joint. Keep up with your orthopedic surgeon's follow-up appointments to keep an eye on the health and function of your joint. During these consultations, your surgeon can detect any possible problems early on and make recommendations for continued care.

To keep your joints supple and your muscles strong, mix low-impact activities into your program. Exercises like swimming, cycling, or light yoga can support the preservation of joint mobility without overtaxing the surgical site. Steer clear of sports or high-impact activities that could exacerbate joint wear and injury.

To lessen the strain on your joints and lower the chance of problems, maintain a healthy weight. The health of your joints and general body is supported by a well-balanced diet full of nutrients including calcium, vitamin D, and omega-3 fatty acids. If you smoke, you should think about giving it up since it might slow down the healing process and raise your risk of complications following joint replacement surgery.

Modifications To Lifestyle For Joint Health

A major factor in the long-term effectiveness of your joint replacement surgery is changing your lifestyle. Make an effort to eat a balanced diet rich in whole grains, lean meats, fruits, and vegetables. These meals offer vital nutrients that promote general healing and joint health.

Include frequent exercise in your regimen to increase general flexibility and strengthen the muscles surrounding the joint. Walking, swimming, and cycling are low-impact exercises that improve cardiovascular health and physical fitness without straining the joints. Steer clear of extended periods of idleness as this may exacerbate joint stiffness and soreness.

Maintain proper body mechanics and posture to lessen the load on your newly formed joint when doing daily tasks. Reduce repetitive stress and promote correct alignment by using ergonomic equipment and furniture. Use cold packs and elevate the afflicted limb if you have joint pain or swelling in order to lessen inflammation and accelerate healing.

Athletics And Exercise Following Rehabilitation

After joint replacement surgery, returning to sports and physical activity needs careful thought and discussion with your healthcare team.

Start with low-impact sports like golfing or swimming, which improve muscular strength and cardiovascular fitness while putting little strain on the joints.

As your strength and confidence grow, gradually reintroduce more strenuous activities like hiking or tennis.

Pay attention to your body's cues and refrain from doing anything that could hurt or cause discomfort at the surgical site. To lessen the chance of harm and extend the life of your replacement joint, use the right technique and safety equipment.

See your physical therapist or orthopedic surgeon before engaging in contact sports or other repetitive impact activities.

They can offer advice on how to protect your joints and avoid issues by changing your technique or selecting different workouts.

After joint replacement surgery, you can resume an active and rewarding lifestyle by progressively increasing your level of activity and taking the necessary precautions.

CHAPTER SEVEN

OTHER MEDICAL SUGGESTIONS AND THERAPIES

Alternatives To Surgery For Joint Pain

Without requiring invasive procedures, non-surgical treatments provide effective alternatives for controlling joint pain and enhancing mobility. These choices use a variety of therapy modalities to reduce pain and improve joint function.

Alternatives To Physical Therapy

Physical therapy offers specific exercises and methods to strengthen surrounding muscles, increase range of motion, and lessen discomfort. In order to improve mobility and function, therapists develop personalized regimens that target individual joint concerns and incorporate stretches, low-impact exercises, and manual treatments. Patients gain from carefully monitored sessions that get harder over time, supporting overall wellness and long-term joint health.

Pharmaceutical and Injectable Treatments

Nonsteroidal anti-inflammatory medications (NSAIDs) are one type of medication that helps control pain and inflammation related to joint disorders. They are frequently used with injectable treatments like hyaluronic acid or corticosteroids.

Corticosteroid injections quickly reduce pain and swelling by injecting anti-inflammatory drugs straight into the joint. Injections of hyaluronic acid improve joint mobility and lower friction by acting as lubricants and shock absorbers.

Methods In Regenerative Medicine

The goal of regenerative medicine is to restore damaged tissues and encourage regeneration by utilizing the body's inherent healing abilities. Injecting concentrated platelets from the patient's own blood into the joint is one method used in platelet-rich plasma (PRP) therapy. Prolotherapy provides a non-surgical means of improving joint health and function by inducing tissue healing and lowering inflammation.

Complementary Medicine For Bone Health

Integrative therapies aim to maximize joint health by combining alternative and traditional medical treatments.

These could include mind-body practices like yoga or meditation, nutritional counseling, chiropractic adjustments, and acupuncture. Integrative therapies seek to improve joint function, lessen pain, and improve overall quality of life by treating the full individual.

CHAPTER EIGHT

IMPACT ON EMOTIONS AND PSYCHOLOGY

Handling Emotional Difficulties

Patients undergoing joint replacement surgery may experience a range of emotions. Before the surgery, it's common to feel nervous, unclear, or even overwhelmed.

Recognizing your emotions and accepting that they are real is the first step toward managing these emotional difficulties.

Speaking with loved ones or support groups about their problems can be beneficial for many patients. This promotes empathy and understanding in addition to releasing emotional tension.

Options For Counseling And Support Systems

A robust support network is essential when undergoing a joint replacement. This includes close relatives and friends as well as medical experts who can offer both practical and emotional support.

In addition to talking to a therapist or attending support groups, counseling alternatives provide more ways to properly manage emotions.

These tools offer a secure setting for talking about anxieties, concerns, and any emotional roadblocks experienced both before and after surgery.

Post-Surgery Mental Health Considerations

Patients frequently feel a range of emotions following joint replacement surgery, such as relief, frustration, or even disappointment.

Acknowledging these emotions and taking proactive measures to address them is part of managing mental health during recovery.

This can be going to counseling sessions on a regular basis, using relaxation techniques, or taking part in activities that support mental health.

Patients who prioritize their mental health can improve their entire experience of rehabilitation and keep a positive attitude toward their advancement.

Community Resources And Peer Assistance

An important part of the mental healing process following joint replacement surgery is peer support. Making connections with people who have experienced comparable operations can offer insightful information, support, and useful coping strategies.

Community resources provide a forum for patients to share their stories, ask questions, and get support from people who really understand their path. Examples of these resources are internet forums and local support groups.

Keeping An Optimistic Attitude

Sustaining an optimistic mindset during the recuperation phase is crucial for general welfare. This entails highlighting minor victories, establishing reasonable objectives, and acknowledging any progress, no matter how slow.

Positivity can also be fostered by engaging in self-care, mindfulness, and gratitude practices. Patients can more easily and confidently overcome the emotional obstacles of joint replacement surgery by developing resilience and optimism.

CHAPTER NINE

COMMON QUESTIONS AND ANSWERS

What is the procedure known as joint replacement? Surgery for joint replacement involves replacing a broken joint with an artificial implant, usually composed of ceramic, metal, or plastic.

It is frequently used to reduce pain and increase mobility in joints that have been severely injured or afflicted by arthritis.

Although elbows, ankles, shoulders, and hips are the most often replaced joints, this procedure can also be used to treat other joints.

Is Joint Replacement Surgery Right for Me? Typically, patients who are candidates for joint replacement surgery have excruciating joint pain, stiffness, and edema that does not go away with conservative measures like medicine or physical therapy.

To decide whether surgery is the best course of action for you, your doctor will assess the degree of joint damage as well as your general health.

What Perils and Difficulties Exist? Risks associated with joint replacement surgery include anesthetic responses, blood clots, and infection.

Nerve injury, implant loosening, and joint dislocation are examples of specific problems. During the procedure, your surgeon will go over these risks with you and take precautions to reduce them.

How Much Time Is Needed for Joint Replacement Surgery? The length of the procedure varies based on the replaced joint and personal circumstances. It usually takes a few hours. There are differences in healing times as well; a full recovery usually takes several months.

What Can I Anticipate From My Rehab? Following an initial hospital stay for joint replacement surgery, patients must undergo physical therapy and rehabilitation to restore strength and mobility. Initially common, pain and discomfort gradually lessen as the joint recovers.

Timetable For Recuperation And Expectations

Following joint replacement surgery, recovery is usually broken down into phases:

Instant Post-Surgery (Hospitalization): Following surgery, you'll need to spend a few days in the hospital to recuperate. During this time, it's critical to start physical therapy, manage pain, and take care of wounds.

First Few Weeks: You'll resume physical therapy following discharge and progressively improve your level of exercise. Daily activities like dressing and taking a shower may require your aid.

First Three Months: To regain strength and range of motion, physical treatment is intensified. You'll experience less pain and swelling and start to feel more at ease using the joint.

Three to Six Months: By this point, the majority of patients have shown a noticeable improvement in their joint function. The goals of physical therapy are to increase flexibility and endurance.

Six Months and Up Many patients resume their regular activities in six months, but it may take up to a year to fully recover. Long-term success requires consistent exercise and follow-up visits.

Going Back To Work And Daily Schedule

Following joint replacement surgery, the following variables must be met before returning to work and daily activities:

Type of Job: Compared to physically demanding employment, sedentary jobs may allow for an earlier return to work.

Recovery Progress: When you can return to work your daily routines depend on your ability to do jobs safely and comfortably.

Physical Therapy: Adhering to the prescribed physical therapy regimen facilitates a seamless return to regular activities and speeds up healing.

Mobility And Travel Considerations

After joint replacement surgery, meticulous planning is necessary for mobility and travel:

Early Post-Surgery Phase: Steer clear of vigorous activities and long-distance travel to promote recovery and avoid problems.

Speak with Your Surgeon: Before booking any travel, speak with your surgeon to make sure it's safe given your level of recuperation.

movement Aids: To help with movement in the early phases of rehabilitation, think about utilizing canes or walkers.

Observational Care And Medical Visits

Monitoring recovery and resolving any issues requires follow-up care:

Post-Operative Visits: Schedule regular visits with your surgeon to evaluate a range of motion, control pain, and monitor recovery.

Check-ins for Physical Therapy: Ongoing physical therapy sessions guarantee continued improvement and handle any mobility problems.

Long-term Monitoring: To evaluate the longevity of the implant and the state of the joint, yearly examinations are advised.

Meeting The Needs For Social And Family Support

Having the support of friends and family is crucial while recovering:

First Support: Helping with everyday tasks can make the journey home easier in the first few days following surgery.

Emotional Support: Getting help and understanding from family and friends is crucial for overcoming the obstacles associated with rehabilitation.

Support through Education: Encouraging family members to become knowledgeable about the healing process enables them to offer suitable help and encouragement.

In order to promote a more seamless recovery and enhanced quality of life, these guidelines are intended to provide patients with a realistic picture of what to anticipate both before and after joint replacement surgery.

www.ingramcontent.com/pod-product-compliance
Lightning Source LLC
Chambersburg PA
CBHW071842210526
45479CB00001B/257